Real Food for Pregnancy Cookbook

Optimising Nutrition for a Healthy Pregnancy Journey

David Lynch

Table of Contents

Introduction: Why Real Food Matters during Pregnancy

As the saying goes, "you are what you eat," and during pregnancy, this couldn't be truer. What a mother-to-be puts into her body has a direct impact on the health and development of her growing baby. Real food, that is, whole, unprocessed, nutrient-dense foods, can make all the difference in promoting a healthy pregnancy and a healthy baby.

Let me tell you about Sarah, a woman who was struggling with fertility for years. She tried everything from fertility treatments to changing her lifestyle, but nothing seemed to work. It wasn't until she started focusing on eating real, whole foods that she finally conceived. During her pregnancy, Sarah continued to prioritise real food, and she noticed a significant difference in her energy levels, mood, and overall well-being.

Sarah's experience is not unique. Many women have reported improved fertility, easier pregnancies, and healthier babies when they adopt a real food diet. In this book, we'll explore why real food matters during pregnancy and how it can make a positive impact on both mother and baby.

Pregnancy is a critical time in a woman's life, as her body is tasked with growing and nurturing a developing baby. A healthy diet during this time is essential to ensure that both mother and baby are receiving the necessary nutrients for optimal growth and development. However, with so much conflicting information about what to eat and what to avoid, it can be challenging to know where to start.

This is where the concept of real food comes in. Real food refers to whole, unprocessed foods that are rich in nutrients and free from additives, preservatives, and artificial ingredients. Think fresh fruits and vegetables, whole grains, lean protein, and healthy fats like nuts and seeds.

When it comes to pregnancy, real food matters for several reasons. First and foremost, it provides essential nutrients that are crucial for foetal development. For example, folate is necessary for proper neural tube development, and calcium is needed for bone growth. Eating a diet rich in real, whole foods can help ensure that these and other vital nutrients are readily available to support a healthy pregnancy.

Real food can also help prevent complications during pregnancy, such as gestational diabetes and preeclampsia. A diet high in processed foods and sugar has been linked to an increased risk of these conditions, while a diet rich in whole foods can help regulate blood sugar and blood pressure levels.

But perhaps the most compelling reason to prioritise real food during pregnancy is its impact on the long-term health of the baby. Research suggests that a mother's diet during pregnancy can influence her child's risk of chronic diseases later in life.

 Now, back to Sarah. She had been trying to conceive for years and was becoming increasingly frustrated with her lack of success. She had tried everything from fertility treatments to changing her lifestyle, but nothing seemed to work. That's when she started to focus on eating real, whole foods.

Sarah began to prioritise nutrient-dense foods like leafy greens, whole grains, and lean protein. She cut back on processed foods and sugar, and she noticed a significant difference in her energy levels, mood, and overall well-being. After a few months of following this real food approach, Sarah discovered that she was pregnant.

Throughout her pregnancy, Sarah continued to prioritise real food, knowing that it was essential for the health of her growing baby. She found that eating a diet rich in whole foods helped her manage her weight, reduce her risk of gestational diabetes, and support her baby's healthy development.

In conclusion, eating real food during pregnancy is crucial for both the mother's and baby's health. A diet rich in whole, unprocessed foods provides essential nutrients, can help prevent complications, and may even influence the long-term health of the baby. As Sarah's story illustrates, making the switch to real food can make all the difference in promoting a healthy pregnancy and a healthy baby.

Chapter 1: The Basics of Real Food Nutrition for Pregnancy

Hello, I'm excited to introduce the first chapter of the book. "This chapter is titled "The Basics of Real Food Nutrition for Pregnancy," and it lays the foundation for the rest of the book by introducing the concept of "real food" and its importance for the health of both mother and baby during pregnancy.

The chapter begins by discussing Understanding Macros and Micronutrients
Building a Balanced Plate
Common Nutrient Deficiencies during Pregnancy

 The chapter also discuss the current state of nutrition advice for pregnant women, which often emphasises calorie counting and the avoidance of certain foods. This is approach is flawed because it fails to consider the nutrient density of foods and can lead to deficiencies in important vitamins and minerals.

Let's talk about the concept of "real food," I defines it as "nutrient-dense, unprocessed or minimally processed, whole foods." Real food, is the key to a healthy pregnancy because it provides the nutrients necessary for foetal development and supports the health of the mother.

As you go on, the chapter goes on to discuss specific nutrients that are particularly important during pregnancy, including protein, fat, and carbohydrates.

In addition to discussing specific nutrients, emphasis is made on the importance of a balanced and varied diet. She provides a list of "superfoods" that are particularly beneficial during pregnancy, such as liver, eggs, and dark leafy greens.

Overall, this chapter provides a valuable introduction to the principles of real food nutrition for pregnancy. By emphasising the importance of nutrient-dense foods and a balanced diet, I also provided a refreshing alternative to the calorie counting and food avoidance that are often promoted during pregnancy. As someone who cares about my women's health and the health of their future baby, I found this chapter to be both informative and empowering.

Understanding Macros and Micronutrients

Macronutrients and micronutrients are crucial for the healthy development of a foetus during pregnancy. Macronutrients, including carbohydrates, proteins, and fats, are required in large amounts, while micronutrients, such as vitamins and minerals, are needed in smaller quantities. We will delve into the importance of macronutrients and micronutrients during pregnancy.

Carbohydrates are the primary source of energy for the body. During pregnancy, the body requires additional energy to support the growing foetus. Therefore, pregnant women should consume an adequate amount of carbohydrates to meet their energy requirements. Carbohydrates are found in foods such as bread, rice, pasta, fruits, and vegetables. Whole grains, fruits, and vegetables are a better source of carbohydrates compared to processed foods. Processed foods may contain high amounts of sugar and are low in fibre, which may lead to an unhealthy weight gain during pregnancy. It's important for pregnant women to choose complex carbohydrates, such as whole grains, fruits, and vegetables, over simple carbohydrates like processed foods and sugary drinks. Complex carbohydrates are rich in fiber, which helps regulate blood sugar levels and prevent constipation, a common problem during pregnancy.

Proteins are essential for the growth and repair of body tissues. During pregnancy, the body requires additional protein to support the growth and development of the foetus. Pregnant women should consume around

75-100 grams of protein per day. Good sources of protein include lean meat, fish, eggs, dairy products, and plant-based sources such as beans, lentils, and tofu. It is essential to consume a variety of protein sources to obtain all the essential amino acids required for fetal growth and development. While animal sources of protein like meat and dairy are excellent sources, plant-based sources like beans, lentils, and tofu are also a great option for pregnant women. Plant-based proteins are typically lower in saturated fats and higher in fibre, which can be beneficial for maternal and foetal health.

Fats are also an important source of energy during pregnancy. Fats play a crucial role in the development of the foetal nervous system and brain. Pregnant women should consume healthy fats, such as unsaturated fats found in nuts, seeds, and vegetable oils, and limit their intake of saturated fats found in high-fat dairy products, meat, and processed foods. Omega-3 fatty acids, found in fish and some plant sources such as flaxseeds, are particularly important during pregnancy. Omega-3 fatty acids have been linked to improved foetal brain development and a reduced risk of preterm birth.

Micronutrients are required in smaller quantities compared to macronutrients but are no less important during pregnancy. Micronutrients play a crucial role in the healthy development of the fetus and the maintenance of maternal health. Below are some important micronutrients during pregnancy.

Folate is a B-vitamin that is essential for foetal neural tube development. Neural tube defects can occur in the early stages of pregnancy before a woman even knows she is pregnant. Therefore, it is essential for women who are trying to conceive or are in their early stages of pregnancy to consume adequate amounts of folate. Good sources of folate include leafy green vegetables, citrus fruits, beans, and fortified cereals.

Iron is required for the formation of red blood cells and the transportation of oxygen throughout the body. During pregnancy, the body requires additional iron to support the growth and development of the fetus. Pregnant women should consume around 27 milligrams of iron per day. Good sources of iron include red meat, poultry, fish, beans, and fortified cereals.

Calcium is essential for the development of strong bones and teeth. Pregnant women should consume around 1000 milligrams of calcium per day. Good sources of calcium include dairy products, fortified plant-based milks, and leafy green vegetables.

Vitamin D is essential for the absorption of calcium and the development of strong bones and teeth. Vitamin D is produced by the body when the skin is exposed to sunlight. However, pregnant women may require additional vitamin D if they have limited sun exposure. Good dietary sources of vitamin D include fatty fish, fortified milk, and fortified cereals.

Vitamin C is essential for the formation of collagen, a protein that is required for the development of skin, cartilage, and bones. Vitamin C also aids in the absorption of iron from plant-based sources, which is especially important for pregnant women who may be at risk of iron deficiency anaemia. Good sources of vitamin C include citrus fruits, berries, kiwi, and vegetables such as bell peppers and broccoli.

Micronutrients: In addition to the micronutrients discussed above, other important micronutrients during pregnancy include zinc, which is required for foetal growth and development, and iodine, which is essential for proper thyroid function and brain development. Pregnant women should aim to consume a balanced diet that includes a variety of nutrient-dense foods to ensure they are meeting their micronutrient needs.

Prenatal supplements: Even with a healthy diet, it can be challenging to meet all nutrient needs during pregnancy. Prenatal supplements can help fill in nutrient gaps and ensure that pregnant women are receiving adequate amounts of important vitamins and minerals. However, it's important to consult with a healthcare provider before starting any supplement regimen, as some supplements can interact with medications or cause adverse effects if taken in excessive amounts.

In summary, a healthy diet that includes a balance of macronutrients and micronutrients is essential for maternal and foetal health during pregnancy. By choosing a variety of nutrient-dense foods and consulting with a healthcare provider or registered dietitian, pregnant women can ensure that they are meeting their nutrient needs and supporting the healthy development of their foetuses.

In conclusion, macronutrients and micronutrients play a crucial role in the healthy development of a foetus during pregnancy. It is essential for pregnant women to consume a balanced diet that includes an adequate amount of carbohydrates, proteins, and fats, as well as important micronutrients such as folate, iron, calcium, vitamin D, and vitamin C. Eating a variety of nutrient-dense foods, such as whole grains, lean proteins, fruits, and vegetables, can help ensure that pregnant women and their foetuses receive the necessary nutrients for optimal health. Additionally, consulting with a healthcare provider or a registered dietitian can help pregnant women tailor their diets to their individual needs and ensure that they are meeting their nutrient requirements.

Building a Balanced Plate

Eating a balanced diet is important for everyone, but it is especially crucial during pregnancy. When you are pregnant, your body needs extra nutrients to support your growing baby. A balanced plate can help ensure that you and your baby are getting the nutrients you need for a healthy pregnancy. In this book, we will explore how to build a balanced plate during pregnancy.

First, it is important to understand what a balanced plate looks like. A balanced plate includes a variety of foods from different food groups. These food groups include:

Fruits and vegetables: Fruits and vegetables are a great source of vitamins, minerals, and fibre. Aim to include a variety of colours in your diet to get a range of nutrients. Try to include at least 2 cups of fruit and 2.5 cups of vegetables per day.

Grains: Grains are an important source of carbohydrates, which provide energy for your body. Choose whole grains, such as brown rice, whole wheat bread, and quinoa, which are higher in fibre and nutrients than refined grains. Aim to include 6-8 ounces of grains per day.

Protein: Protein is important for building and repairing tissues in your body, including your baby's. Good sources of protein include lean meats, poultry, fish, beans, and tofu. Aim to include 6-8 ounces of protein per day.

Dairy: Dairy products are a good source of calcium, which is important for building strong bones and teeth. Choose low-fat or fat-free options, such as milk, cheese, and yoghourt. Aim to include 3 cups of dairy per day.

Fats: Fats are important for providing energy and helping your body absorb certain vitamins. Choose healthy fats, such as those found in nuts, seeds, avocados, and olive oil. Limit saturated and trans fats, which can increase your risk of heart disease.

Now that we know what a balanced plate looks like, let's explore how to put it into practice during pregnancy.

Start with a base of fruits and vegetables. Aim to fill half of your plate with fruits and vegetables. This will provide a range of nutrients, including vitamins, minerals, and fibre. Try to include a variety of colours to get a range of nutrients.

Add a serving of grains. Grains provide carbohydrates, which provide energy for your body. Choose whole grains, such as brown rice, whole wheat bread, and quinoa, which are higher in fiber and nutrients than refined grains. Aim to include 1-2 servings of grains per meal.

Include a serving of protein. Protein is important for building and repairing tissues in your body, including your baby's. Good sources of protein include lean meats, poultry, fish, beans, and tofu. Aim to include 1-2 servings of protein per meal.

Include a serving of dairy. Dairy products are a good source of calcium, which is important for building strong bones and teeth. Choose low-fat or fat-free options, such as milk, cheese, and yoghourt. Aim to include 1-2 servings of dairy per day.

Add healthy fats. Fats are important for providing energy and helping your body absorb certain vitamins. Choose healthy fats, such as those found in nuts, seeds, avocados, and olive oil. Limit saturated and trans fats, which can increase your risk of heart disease. Aim to include a small serving of healthy fats in each meal.

In addition to building a balanced plate, there are some specific nutrients that are particularly important during pregnancy.

Folic acid: Folic acid is important for the development of the neural tube, which forms the baby's brain and spinal cord. It is recommended that women who are planning to become pregnant take 400-800 micrograms of folic acid daily, and that pregnant women take 600-800 micrograms per day.

Iron: Iron is necessary for the production of haemoglobin, which carries oxygen in the blood. During pregnancy, a woman's blood volume increases to support the growing foetus, so she needs more iron. Pregnant women should aim to get at least 27 milligrams of iron per day.

Calcium: Calcium is important for the development of the baby's bones and teeth, and for maintaining the mother's bone health. Pregnant women should aim to get 1,000-1,300 milligrams of calcium per day.

Vitamin D: Vitamin D is important for the absorption of calcium and for the development of the baby's bones and teeth. Pregnant women should aim to get at least 600-800 international units (IU) of vitamin D per day.

Omega-3 fatty acids: Omega-3 fatty acids are important for the development of the baby's brain and eyes. Pregnant women should aim to get at least 200-300 milligrams of DHA (a type of omega-3 fatty acid) per day.

Protein: Protein is important for the growth and development of the baby's tissues, and for maintaining the mother's health. Pregnant women should aim to get 75-100 grams of protein per day, depending on their weight.

It's important for pregnant women to talk to their healthcare provider about their individual nutrient needs and to take a prenatal vitamin to help ensure they are getting all the necessary nutrients for a healthy pregnancy.

Dehydration can be a significant concern during exercise, especially for pregnant women who need to maintain their fluid balance for their own health and the health of their developing foetus. During exercise, the body loses fluids through sweating, and if these fluids are not replenished, it can lead to dehydration.

Dehydration during pregnancy can cause a variety of problems, including headaches, dizziness, cramping, and fatigue. It can also increase the risk of preterm labour and low birth weight.

To prevent dehydration during exercise, pregnant women should drink plenty of fluids before, during, and after exercise. It's recommended that pregnant women drink at least 8-10 cups (64-80 ounces) of water per day, and even more if they are exercising.

In addition to water, pregnant women can also consume fluids that contain electrolytes, such as sports drinks or coconut water, to help replenish the minerals lost through sweating.

It's also important for pregnant women to listen to their bodies during exercise and to avoid pushing themselves too hard. They should take breaks as needed, and avoid exercising in hot or humid environments, which can increase the risk of dehydration.

Overall, by staying well-hydrated during exercise and throughout pregnancy, women can help ensure the health and well-being of themselves and their developing foetus.

Chapter 2: Meal Planning for a Healthy Pregnancy

Congratulations on your pregnancy! One of the most important things you can do for yourself and your growing baby is to maintain a healthy diet throughout your pregnancy. Eating a balanced diet that is rich in nutrients can help ensure that your baby develops properly and that you stay healthy and energized during this exciting time.

In this chapter, we will discuss the basics of meal planning for a healthy pregnancy. We will cover important nutrients that you and your baby need, foods to avoid, and tips for making healthy and delicious meals. Whether you are an experienced cook or a novice in the kitchen, this chapter will provide you with the information and tools you need to make sure you are eating well during your pregnancy.

How to Plan Meals with Real Food

Planning meals with real food can be beneficial for maintaining a healthy diet, especially during pregnancy. Here are some steps to follow when planning meals with real food:

Start by reviewing your weekly schedule: Consider your schedule for the week ahead, including work, school, appointments, and social engagements. This will help you determine how many meals you need to plan for, and when you will have time to prepare them.

Make a list of healthy ingredients: Once you have an idea of how many meals you need to plan for, make a list of healthy ingredients that you would like to include in your meals. Focus on nutrient-dense whole foods, such as fruits, vegetables, whole grains, lean proteins, and healthy fats.

Choose recipes: Look for recipes that incorporate the ingredients on your list. Consider your dietary preferences, any food allergies or intolerances, and any specific nutritional needs that you have.

Plan your meals: Use a meal planning template or calendar to plan out your meals for the week. Be sure to include breakfast, lunch, dinner, and snacks. Aim to balance each meal with a variety of nutrient-dense whole foods.

Prepare your meals: Once you have planned your meals, make a grocery list and purchase the ingredients you need. Set aside time each day or week to prepare your meals in advance, so that you have healthy options readily available.

Benefits of planning meals with real food include:

Improved nutrition: Planning meals with real food can help you to consume a variety of nutrient-dense whole foods, which can improve your overall nutrition.

Time and money savings: By planning your meals in advance, you can save time and money by reducing food waste and avoiding last-minute trips to the grocery store or takeout.

Increased energy and focus: Eating a balanced diet of real food can provide you with sustained energy throughout the day and improve mental focus.

Healthier weight: Eating a balanced diet of real food can help you maintain a healthy weight and reduce the risk of chronic diseases.

Overall, planning meals with real food can be a helpful tool for maintaining a healthy diet during pregnancy and beyond.

Sample Meal Plans for Each Trimester

During pregnancy, it's important to eat a well-balanced diet to ensure that both the mother and the baby get all the necessary nutrients. The dietary requirements change during each trimester of pregnancy, and here are some sample meal plans for each trimester:

First Trimester

During the first trimester, many women experience nausea and vomiting, so it's important to eat small, frequent meals throughout the day to avoid an empty stomach. It's also important to stay hydrated by drinking plenty of water and fluids.

Sample Meal Plan:

Breakfast:

Whole grain toast with almond butter and sliced banana
Yoghourt with granola and berries
Herbal tea or decaf coffee
Mid-morning snack:

Apple slices with almond butter
Hard-boiled egg
Carrots and hummus
Lunch:

Grilled chicken salad with mixed greens, avocado, and a light vinaigrette
Quinoa salad with roasted vegetables and feta cheese
Bean burrito with whole wheat tortilla and salsa
Afternoon snack:

Trail mix with nuts, seeds, and dried fruit
Greek yoghourt with honey and walnuts
Cheese and crackers
Dinner:

Baked salmon with roasted sweet potatoes and broccoli
Lentil soup with whole grain bread

Stir-fry with brown rice, tofu, and vegetables
Second Trimester

During the second trimester, the nausea usually subsides, and the baby starts to grow rapidly. It's important to consume more calories and protein during this stage.

Sample Meal Plan:

Breakfast:

Whole grain waffles with almond butter and sliced banana
Greek yoghourt with granola and berries
Green smoothie with spinach, banana, and almond milk
Mid-morning snack:

Fresh fruit salad
Cottage cheese with pineapple
Hummus and whole grain pita
Lunch:

Grilled chicken sandwich with avocado and whole grain bread
Whole wheat pasta with tomato sauce and grilled vegetables
Falafel wrap with hummus and tzatziki sauce
Afternoon snack:

Whole grain crackers with cheese and apple slices
Peanut butter and jelly sandwich
Homemade energy bars
Dinner:

Grilled steak with roasted sweet potatoes and green beans
Baked chicken with quinoa and roasted vegetables
Vegetarian chilli with brown rice and avocado
Third Trimester

During the third trimester, the baby's growth continues, and the mother's body prepares for labour and delivery. It's important to eat foods that provide plenty of energy and nutrients.

Sample Meal Plan:

Breakfast:

Oatmeal with nuts and berries
Whole grain toast with avocado and scrambled eggs
Smoothie bowl with frozen berries and Greek yoghourt
Mid-morning snack:

Rice cakes with almond butter and banana slices
Hard-boiled egg with whole grain crackers
Fruit and yoghourt parfait
Lunch:

Grilled salmon with quinoa and mixed vegetables
Turkey and cheese wrap with hummus and vegetables
Lentil soup with whole grain bread
Afternoon snack:

Carrots and celery with hummus
Banana and peanut butter smoothie
Energy balls with nuts and dates
Dinner:

Roasted chicken with sweet potato and green beans
Grilled shrimp with quinoa and mixed vegetables
Baked tofu with brown rice and steamed broccoli
It's important to note that each woman's dietary needs are different, and these sample meal plans are not intended to replace the advice of a healthcare provider. It's always best to consult with a healthcare provider for individualised dietary recommendations during pregnancy.

Tips for Managing Cravings and Nausea

Pregnancy can come with a variety of symptoms, including cravings and nausea. Here are some tips for managing both:

Managing Cravings:

Choose healthy options: Instead of giving into every craving, try to choose healthier options. For example, if you're craving something sweet, reach for a piece of fruit instead of candy.

Plan your meals: Try to plan your meals and snacks ahead of time to help curb cravings. Make sure you're eating regularly throughout the day to avoid getting too hungry, which can lead to stronger cravings.

Stay hydrated: Drinking plenty of water can help reduce cravings. Sometimes thirst can be mistaken for hunger or cravings, so make sure you're getting enough water throughout the day.

Keep busy: Distract yourself when you feel a craving coming on. Try going for a walk, calling a friend, or doing something you enjoy to take your mind off the craving.

Managing Nausea:

Eat small, frequent meals: Eating smaller, more frequent meals can help keep your blood sugar levels stable and reduce nausea. Try to eat something every 2-3 hours.

Avoid trigger foods: Certain foods may trigger nausea, so try to avoid them if possible. Common triggers include spicy or fatty foods, caffeine, and strong smells.

Stay hydrated: Dehydration can make nausea worse, so it's important to stay hydrated. Sip water or ginger ale throughout the day to help settle your stomach.

Get plenty of rest: Fatigue can make nausea worse, so make sure you're getting plenty of rest. Take naps during the day if you need to, and try to get a full night's sleep.

Remember, it's important to talk to your healthcare provider if you're experiencing severe or persistent cravings or nausea during pregnancy. They can help you develop a plan to manage your symptoms and ensure the health of you and your baby.

Chapter 3: Real Food Recipes for a Nourishing Pregnancy

In this chapter, we will explore a variety of real food recipes that are perfect for supporting a healthy and nourishing pregnancy. Eating a balanced and nutritious diet is essential during pregnancy, as it not only supports the health of the mother but also the growth and development of the growing baby. These recipes are made with whole, nutrient-dense ingredients that are rich in vitamins, minerals, and antioxidants. They are designed to provide the necessary nutrients to support a healthy pregnancy and ensure optimal foetal development. From breakfast to dinner and snacks in between, these recipes are delicious and easy to prepare, making it easier for pregnant women to make healthy food choices. So, let's dive in and discover some nourishing pregnancy recipes!

Breakfast

A healthy and balanced breakfast is important for pregnant women as it provides essential nutrients and energy for both the mother and the growing foetus.

Breakfast is important for pregnant women for several reasons:

Provides energy: Breakfast is the first meal of the day, and it provides essential nutrients and energy to start the day. For pregnant women, it is important to maintain their energy levels as their bodies are working hard to support the growth and development of their baby.

Prevents morning sickness: Eating a healthy breakfast can help prevent morning sickness, which is a common symptom of pregnancy. Having an empty stomach can aggravate nausea and vomiting, so having a small meal in the morning can help reduce these symptoms.

Maintains blood sugar levels: Pregnancy can cause fluctuations in blood sugar levels, which can lead to gestational diabetes. Eating a healthy breakfast can help maintain stable blood sugar levels and reduce the risk of gestational diabetes.

Provides essential nutrients: A healthy breakfast can provide essential nutrients such as folic acid, iron, calcium, and vitamins. These nutrients are important for the baby's growth and development and can also help prevent birth defects.

Overall, breakfast is an important meal for pregnant women as it provides energy, prevents morning sickness, maintains blood sugar levels, and provides essential nutrients. Pregnant women should aim to have a balanced and nutritious breakfast to support their health and the health of their growing baby.

Here are nutritious breakfast recipes suitable for pregnancy:

Oatmeal with Fruit and Nuts

Ingredients:

1/2 cup rolled oats
1 cup water or milk (dairy or non-dairy)
1/2 cup mixed fresh or frozen fruit (such as berries, sliced bananas, or chopped apples)
1 tablespoon chopped nuts (such as almonds or walnuts)
1 teaspoon honey or maple syrup (optional)

Instructions:

Combine the oats and water or milk in a small pot and bring to a boil. Reduce heat to low and cook, stirring occasionally, for about 5 minutes or until the oats are tender and the mixture has thickened.

Remove from heat and stir in the fruit, nuts, and sweetener (if using).
Serve warm.

Nutrition profile:
This breakfast is rich in fibre from the oats and fruit, as well as healthy
fats and protein from the nuts. It also provides essential vitamins and
minerals such as vitamin C, potassium, and iron from the fruit.

Note:
You can customise this recipe by adding different types of fruit or nuts
depending on your preference and availability. Be sure to choose
unsweetened milk alternatives if you are using non-dairy milk to keep
added sugars to a minimum.

Greek Yoghourt Parfait

Ingredients:

1 cup plain Greek yoghourt
1/2 cup mixed fresh or frozen fruit (such as berries, sliced bananas, or
chopped mango)
1/4 cup granola or muesli
1 tablespoon honey or maple syrup (optional)

Instructions:

In a bowl or glass, layer the yoghourt, fruit, and granola or muesli.
Drizzle with honey or maple syrup (if using).
Serve chilled.

Nutrition profile:
This breakfast is rich in protein and calcium from the Greek yogurt, as
well as fibre and vitamins from the fruit and granola or muesli.

Note:
You can choose low-fat or non-fat Greek yoghourt if you prefer to reduce
your intake of saturated fat. Be sure to read the labels when selecting

granola or muesli, as some brands may contain added sugars or
unhealthy fats.

Veggie Omelette

Ingredients:

2 eggs
1/4 cup chopped vegetables (such as spinach, bell peppers, mushrooms,
or onions)
1 tablespoon olive oil or butter
Salt and pepper to taste

Instructions:

In a bowl, beat the eggs with a fork and season with salt and pepper.
Heat the oil or butter in a small non-stick skillet over medium heat.
Add the vegetables and cook for 2-3 minutes or until they are softened.
Pour the beaten eggs over the vegetables and cook for 2-3 minutes or
until the bottom is set.
Use a spatula to carefully flip the omelette and cook for another 1-2
minutes or until the eggs are fully cooked.
Serve hot.

Nutrition profile:
This breakfast is high in protein from the eggs, as well as vitamins,
minerals, and fibre from the vegetables. The use of olive oil provides
healthy monounsaturated fats.

Note:
You can choose any combination of vegetables for the omelette based on
your taste preferences. Be sure to cook the eggs thoroughly to reduce the
risk of foodborne illness.

Peanut Butter Banana Toast

Ingredients:

1 slice whole wheat bread
1 tablespoon natural peanut butter
1/2 medium banana, sliced

Instructions:

Toast the bread until crispy.
Spread the peanut butter evenly on the toast.
Top with sliced banana.
Serve immediately.
Nutrition profile:
This breakfast is high in fibre and protein from the whole wheat bread
and peanut butter, as well as vitamins and minerals from the banana.

Note:
Be sure to choose natural peanut butter without added sugars or oils to
keep the recipe healthy. You can also add some chia or flax seeds for an
extra boost of omega-3 fatty acids.

Blueberry Chia Seed Pudding

Ingredients:

1/4 cup chia seeds
1 cup unsweetened almond milk
1/2 cup fresh or frozen blueberries
1 tablespoon honey or maple syrup (optional)
1/4 teaspoon vanilla extract (optional)

Instructions:

In a jar or bowl, combine the chia seeds, almond milk, honey or maple
syrup (if using), and vanilla extract (if using). Stir well.
Add the blueberries and stir gently.
Cover and refrigerate overnight or for at least 2 hours.
Serve chilled.

Nutrition profile:
This breakfast is high in fibre, protein, and healthy fats from the chia
seeds, as well as antioxidants and vitamins from the blueberries.

Note:
You can use any type of milk or milk alternative for this recipe. If you
prefer a smoother texture, you can blend the pudding ingredients (except
the blueberries) in a blender before adding the fruit.

Sweet Potato and Black Bean Breakfast Burrito

Ingredients:

1 small sweet potato, peeled and diced
1/4 cup black beans, drained and rinsed
2 eggs, beaten
1 tablespoon olive oil
1/4 teaspoon chilli powder
Salt and pepper to taste
1 whole wheat tortilla

Instructions:

Heat the olive oil in a small non-stick skillet over medium heat.
Add the sweet potato and chilli powder and cook for 5-7 minutes or until
the sweet potato is tender.
Add the black beans and cook for another 2-3 minutes or until heated
through.
Pour the beaten eggs over the sweet potato and black bean mixture and
cook for 2-3 minutes or until the eggs are set.
Season with salt and pepper to taste.
Spoon the egg mixture onto a tortilla and roll up.
Serve hot.

Nutrition profile:
This breakfast is high in fibre and protein from the sweet potato and
black beans, as well as vitamins and minerals from the eggs.

Note:
You can customise the filling by using different types of beans or vegetables. You can also add some salsa or avocado for extra flavour and nutrition. Be sure to choose a whole wheat tortilla for added fibre.

Greek Yoghourt Parfait

Ingredients:

1 cup plain Greek yoghourt
1/2 cup mixed fresh berries (such as blueberries, strawberries, and raspberries)
1/4 cup granola
1 tablespoon honey

Instructions:

In a small bowl, mix together the Greek yoghourt and honey.
In a separate bowl, mix together the mixed berries.
Layer the Greek yoghourt mixture, mixed berries, and granola in a glass or jar.
Serve immediately.

Nutrition profile:
This breakfast is high in protein from the Greek yoghourt and fibre from the berries and granola. It also contains antioxidants and vitamins from the berries.

Note:
You can use any type of fruit or granola you prefer. You can also add some nuts or seeds for an extra crunch.

Spinach and Feta Omelette

Ingredients:

2 eggs
1/2 cup fresh spinach

1/4 cup crumbled feta cheese
1 tablespoon olive oil
Salt and pepper to taste

Instructions:

Beat the eggs in a small bowl.
Heat the olive oil in a non-stick skillet over medium heat.
Add the spinach and cook for 1-2 minutes or until wilted.
Pour the eggs over the spinach and cook for 2-3 minutes or until set.
Sprinkle the feta cheese over the eggs.
Season with salt and pepper to taste.
Fold the omelette in half and serve hot.

Nutrition profile:
This breakfast is high in protein and healthy fats from the eggs and feta
cheese. It also contains vitamins and minerals from the spinach.

Note:
You can add some diced tomatoes or mushrooms to the omelette for
extra flavor and nutrition.

Overnight Oats with Almond Butter and Banana

Ingredients:

1/2 cup rolled oats
1/2 cup unsweetened almond milk
1/2 medium banana, mashed
1 tablespoon almond butter
1 teaspoon honey (optional)
Instructions:

In a jar or bowl, mix together the rolled oats, almond milk, mashed
banana, almond butter, and honey (if using).
Cover and refrigerate overnight or for at least 2 hours.
Serve chilled.

Nutrition profile:
This breakfast is high in fiber and healthy fats from the rolled oats and almond butter, as well as vitamins and minerals from the banana.

Note:
You can use any type of nut butter or milk alternative you prefer. You can also add some cinnamon or vanilla extract for extra flavor. If you prefer a sweeter taste, you can add more honey or maple syrup.

Lunch

Lunch is an important meal during pregnancy because it provides essential nutrients to the mother and the growing baby. The body of a pregnant woman requires extra energy to support the developing fetus and to maintain the mother's health. Lunch is a great opportunity to ensure that the body gets the required nutrients and energy to support the pregnancy.

During pregnancy, the body needs a variety of nutrients, such as protein, iron, calcium, folic acid, and vitamin C. These nutrients are essential for the growth and development of the baby's organs, bones, and muscles. Additionally, the mother's body needs these nutrients to support the increased blood volume, hormone production, and metabolism.

Having a balanced lunch that includes a variety of food groups is important during pregnancy. A healthy lunch should include protein sources like lean meat, fish, beans, or tofu, complex carbohydrates like whole grains, vegetables, fruits, and healthy fats like avocados, nuts, and seeds. This combination of foods will provide the necessary nutrients and energy to support the pregnancy.

Skipping lunch or having a meal that is lacking in essential nutrients can cause problems during pregnancy. It can lead to low birth weight, premature birth, and developmental delays. Additionally, a lack of nutrients can result in fatigue, anaemia, and other health problems for the mother.

It is important to note that pregnant women should avoid certain foods that can be harmful to the baby, such as raw or undercooked meat, fish, and eggs, unpasteurized dairy products, and deli meats. They should also limit their intake of caffeine, alcohol, and processed foods.

In conclusion, lunch is an important meal during pregnancy as it provides essential nutrients and energy to support the growth and development of the baby and the mother's health. Pregnant women should aim for a balanced meal that includes a variety of food groups and avoid foods that can be harmful to the baby. By making healthy choices at lunchtime, pregnant women can support a healthy pregnancy and give their baby the best possible start in life.

Here are some lunch recipes to try out

Grilled Chicken Salad

Ingredients:
1 chicken breast
mixed greens
cherry tomatoes
cucumber
red onion
2 tbsp balsamic vinaigrette
salt and pepper to taste

Recipe:

Grill chicken breast until cooked through
Chop mixed greens, cherry tomatoes, cucumber, and red onion
Toss salad ingredients together with balsamic vinaigrette
Slice chicken and add to salad
Add salt and pepper to taste

Notes: This salad is packed with vitamins and minerals from the mixed greens, tomatoes, and cucumber. Chicken provides protein and iron, which are important nutrients for pregnant women.

Quinoa Stuffed Bell Peppers

Ingredients:
4 bell peppers
1 cup quinoa
1 can black beans, drained and rinsed
1 cup corn
1 tsp cumin
1 tsp chili powder
1/2 cup shredded cheddar cheese
salt and pepper to taste

Recipe:

Preheat oven to 375°F (190°C)
Cut the tops off the bell peppers and remove the seeds and membranes
In a bowl, mix cooked quinoa, black beans, corn, cumin, chili powder,
salt, and pepper
Stuff the bell peppers with the quinoa mixture and place them in a
baking dish
Sprinkle shredded cheese on top of the stuffed bell peppers
Bake for 30-35 minutes or until the cheese is melted and bubbly

Notes: This dish is a good source of plant-based protein, fibre, and iron
from the quinoa and black beans. Bell peppers are also rich in vitamin C,
which helps with iron absorption.

Lentil Soup

Ingredients:
1 cup lentils
1 onion, diced
2 carrots, peeled and diced
2 celery stalks, diced
4 cups vegetable or chicken broth
1 tsp cumin
1 tsp paprika
salt and pepper to taste

Recipe:
Rinse lentils and set aside
In a large pot, sauté onion, carrots, and celery until soft
Add lentils, broth, cumin, paprika, salt, and pepper to the pot
Bring to a boil, then reduce heat and simmer for 25-30 minutes or until
the lentils are tender
Serve hot

Notes: Lentils are a good source of protein, fiber, and iron. They are also
low in fat and calories, making this soup a healthy option for pregnant
women.

Salmon and Sweet Potato

Ingredients:
1 salmon fillet
1 sweet potato, peeled and diced
2 cups spinach
1 tbsp olive oil
salt and pepper to taste

Recipe:
Preheat oven to 400°F (200°C)
Place salmon fillet on a baking sheet and season with salt and pepper
In a separate baking dish, toss sweet potato with olive oil, salt, and
pepper
Bake salmon and sweet potato in the oven for 20-25 minutes or until the
salmon is cooked through and the sweet potato is tender
Serve salmon and sweet potato on a bed of spinach

Notes: Salmon is a good source of omega-3 fatty acids, which are
important for brain and eye development in babies. Sweet potatoes are
rich in vitamins A and C, which help with immune function and foetal
growth.

Greek Yogurt and Fruit Parfait

Ingredients:

1 cup Greek yoghourt
1 cup mixed fresh berries
1/4 cup granola

Recipe:
Layer Greek yoghourt, berries, and granola in a bowl or cup
Repeat until all ingredients are used up
Serve chilled

Notes: Greek yoghourt is a good source of protein and calcium, which are important for foetal development. Berries are rich in antioxidants and fibre, which support a healthy pregnancy.

Chicken Fajita Bowl

Ingredients:
1 chicken breast
1 bell pepper, sliced
1 onion, sliced
1 tbsp olive oil
1 tsp chilli powder
1 tsp cumin
1/2 cup cooked brown rice
1/4 cup black beans, drained and rinsed
1/4 cup shredded cheddar cheese
salt and pepper to taste

Recipe:

Grill or bake chicken breast until cooked through
In a pan, sauté bell pepper and onion in olive oil until tender
Add chilli powder, cumin, salt, and pepper to the pan and mix well
Assemble bowl with cooked brown rice, black beans, sautéed bell pepper and onion mixture, sliced chicken, and shredded cheddar cheese

Notes: This bowl is a good source of protein, fibre, and complex carbohydrates. Brown rice and black beans provide folate and iron, which are important for foetal development.

Veggie Wrap

Ingredients:
1 whole wheat tortilla
1/4 avocado, mashed
1/4 cup hummus
1/4 cup shredded carrots
1/4 cup sliced cucumbers
1/4 cup mixed greens
salt and pepper to taste

Recipe:

Lay tortilla flat
Spread mashed avocado and hummus on the tortilla
Add shredded carrots, sliced cucumbers, and mixed greens
Roll up tortilla and slice in half

Notes: This wrap is packed with nutrients from the vegetables and healthy fats from the avocado. Hummus provides protein and fiber.

Lentil and Spinach Curry

Ingredients:
1 cup lentils
1 onion, diced
2 cloves garlic, minced
2 cups spinach
1 can diced tomatoes
1 tsp turmeric
1 tsp cumin
1 tsp coriander
salt and pepper to taste

Recipe:

Rinse lentils and set aside
In a pan, sauté onion and garlic until soft
Add lentils, canned tomatoes, turmeric, cumin, coriander, salt, and pepper to the pan
Bring to a boil, then reduce heat and simmer for 25-30 minutes or until the lentils are tender
Stir in spinach until wilted
Serve hot with brown rice or naan

Notes: Lentils provide protein, fibre, and iron. Spinach is rich in folate, which is important for foetal development. The spices in this curry provide flavour and antioxidants.

Tuna Salad Sandwich

Ingredients:

2 cans of tuna, drained
1/4 cup mayonnaise
1/4 cup Greek yoghourt
1/4 cup diced celery
1/4 cup diced red onion
1 tablespoon chopped fresh parsley
1 teaspoon Dijon mustard
Salt and pepper to taste

Recipe:

In a medium-sized bowl, combine the drained tuna, mayonnaise, Greek yoghourt, celery, red onion, parsley, and Dijon mustard.
Mix everything together until well combined.
Season with salt and pepper to taste.
Serve the tuna salad on whole wheat bread, mixed greens, or crackers.

Notes: Tuna is a good source of protein and omega-3 fatty acids, which are important for foetal brain and eye development. Greek yoghourt is a healthier alternative to using all mayonnaise, and provides additional protein and calcium. The celery and red onion add flavour and nutrients like vitamin C and fibre.

Dinner

Dinner is an important meal for anyone, including pregnant women. During pregnancy, a woman's body requires extra nutrients to support the growth and development of the foetus, and dinner is an excellent opportunity to consume these nutrients.

Here are some specific reasons why dinner is important during pregnancy:

Provides necessary nutrients: Dinner is an opportunity to consume a balanced meal that includes a variety of nutrients, such as protein, calcium, iron, and folic acid. These nutrients are essential for the growth and development of the foetus, and can help prevent complications such as neural tube defects and low birth weight.

Helps control weight: Eating a nutritious dinner can help prevent excessive weight gain during pregnancy, which can increase the risk of complications such as gestational diabetes, preeclampsia, and caesarean delivery.

Regulates blood sugar: Eating dinner can help regulate blood sugar levels, which is important during pregnancy as high blood sugar levels can lead to gestational diabetes.

Supports sleep: A balanced dinner can help promote better sleep, which is important for both the mother and the developing foetus.

Helps prevent acid reflux: Pregnant women are more susceptible to acid reflux, and eating a light, balanced dinner can help prevent this uncomfortable condition.

Overall, a healthy and balanced dinner is important during pregnancy to ensure that the mother and foetus receive the necessary nutrients for optimal growth and development, and to prevent complications.

Baked Salmon with Quinoa and Roasted Vegetables:

Ingredients:

1 lb salmon fillet
1 cup quinoa
2 cups water
1 small sweet potato, peeled and cubed
1 small zucchini, sliced
1 small red onion, sliced
2 tablespoons olive oil
1 teaspoon dried oregano
Salt and pepper to taste

Instructions:

Preheat the oven to 375°F (190°C).
In a medium pot, bring the water to a boil. Add the quinoa and reduce heat to low. Cover and cook for 15-20 minutes, or until the water is absorbed and the quinoa is fluffy.
Arrange the sweet potato, zucchini, and red onion on a baking sheet. Drizzle with olive oil and sprinkle with oregano, salt, and pepper. Toss to coat.
Place the salmon on top of the vegetables. Season with salt and pepper. Bake for 20-25 minutes, or until the salmon is cooked through and the vegetables are tender.
Serve the salmon and vegetables over the quinoa.

Benefits: Salmon is a great source of omega-3 fatty acids, which are important for foetal brain and eye development. Quinoa is a whole grain that is high in protein, fibre, and essential vitamins and minerals. Sweet potatoes are a good source of vitamin C, which helps the body absorb iron.

Nutrition Profile (per serving):
Calories: 501
Protein: 35g
Fat: 21g
Carbohydrates: 41g
Fiber: 6g

Lentil Soup with Spinach and Tomatoes:

Ingredients:

1 cup dried green lentils
4 cups low-sodium vegetable broth
1 can diced tomatoes, undrained
1 small onion, chopped
2 cloves garlic, minced
2 cups fresh spinach, chopped
1 tablespoon olive oil
1 teaspoon ground cumin
Salt and pepper to taste

Instructions:

In a large pot, heat the olive oil over medium heat. Add the onion and
garlic and sauté for 2-3 minutes, or until the onion is translucent.
Add the lentils, vegetable broth, diced tomatoes, cumin, salt, and pepper
to the pot. Bring to a boil, then reduce heat to low and simmer for 30-40
minutes, or until the lentils are tender.
Add the chopped spinach to the pot and stir until wilted.
Serve the soup hot, with a slice of whole grain bread on the side if
desired.

Benefits: Lentils are high in protein, fibre, and iron, which is important
for pregnant women to prevent anaemia. Spinach is a good source of
folate, which is important for foetal development.

Nutrition Profile (per serving):
Calories: 275

Protein: 15g
Fat: 4g
Carbohydrates: 45g
Fibre: 18g

Grilled Chicken with Roasted Vegetables and Brown Rice:

Ingredients:

4 boneless, skinless chicken breasts
2 cups broccoli florets
2 cups sliced mushrooms
1 small red onion, sliced
2 tablespoons olive oil
1 teaspoon dried thyme
Salt and pepper to taste
2 cups cooked brown rice

Instructions:

Preheat the grill to medium-high heat.
In a large bowl, toss the broccoli, mushrooms, and red onion with olive
oil, thyme, salt, and pepper.
Place the vegetables on a large sheet of aluminium foil and fold up the
edges to create a packet. Place the packet on the grill and cook for 10-15
minutes, or until the vegetables are tender.
Season the chicken breasts with salt and pepper. Grill the chicken for 6-7
minutes per side, or until cooked through.
Serve the chicken and roasted vegetables over the brown rice.

Benefits: Chicken is a good source of protein, and vegetables provide
important vitamins and minerals. Brown rice is a whole grain that is high
in fibre and essential nutrients.

Nutrition Profile (per serving):
Calories: 396
Protein: 33g
Fat: 11g

Carbohydrates: 43g
Fiber: 6g

Turkey Chili with Sweet Potatoes and Black Beans:

Ingredients:

1 lb ground turkey
1 small sweet potato, peeled and cubed
1 can black beans, drained and rinsed
1 can diced tomatoes, undrained
1 small onion, chopped
2 cloves garlic, minced
1 tablespoon chilli powder
1 teaspoon ground cumin
Salt and pepper to taste

Instructions:

In a large pot, cook the ground turkey over medium heat until browned.
Add the sweet potato, black beans, diced tomatoes, onion, garlic, chilli
powder, cumin, salt, and pepper to the pot. Stir to combine.
Bring the chilli to a boil, then reduce heat to low and simmer for 20-30
minutes, or until the sweet potato is tender and the flavours are blended.
Serve the chilli hot, topped with shredded cheese and a dollop of plain
Greek yoghourt if desired.

Benefits: Ground turkey is a lean protein source, and sweet potatoes are
high in vitamin C, folate, and fibre. Black beans are a good source of
protein and fibre.

Nutrition Profile (per serving):
Calories: 313
Protein: 28g
Fat: 9g
Carbohydrates: 30g
Fibre: 8g

Veggie and Tofu Stir Fry:

Ingredients:

1 block extra firm tofu, drained and cubed
2 cups broccoli florets
1 cup sliced mushrooms
1 small red bell pepper, sliced
2 cloves garlic, minced
1 tablespoon soy sauce
1 tablespoon cornstarch
2 tablespoons olive oil
Salt and pepper to taste
2 cups cooked brown rice

Instructions:

In a small bowl, whisk together the soy sauce and cornstarch until smooth.
In a large skillet or wok, heat the olive oil over high heat. Add the tofu and cook for 5-7 minutes, or until browned.
Add the broccoli, mushrooms, red bell pepper, and garlic to the skillet. Stir fry for 5-7 minutes, or until the vegetables are tender.
Pour the soy sauce mixture over the vegetables and tofu. Stir to combine and cook for 1-2 minutes, or until the sauce has thickened.
Serve the stir fry hot, over brown rice.

Benefits: Tofu is a good source of protein and calcium, and vegetables provide important vitamins and minerals. Brown rice is a whole grain that is high in fibre and essential nutrients.

Nutrition Profile (per serving):
Calories: 339
Protein: 16g
Fat: 14g
Carbohydrates: 38g
Fibre: 6g

Baked Sweet Potato with Broccoli and Cheese:

Ingredients:

2 small sweet potatoes
2 cups broccoli florets
1/2 cup shredded cheddar cheese
1 tablespoon olive oil
Salt and pepper to taste

Instructions:

Preheat the oven to 400°F (200°C).
Pierce the sweet potatoes with a fork several times. Rub them with olive oil and sprinkle with salt and pepper.
Place the sweet potatoes on a baking sheet and bake for 40-50 minutes, or until tender.
In the last 10 minutes of baking, place the broccoli florets on the baking sheet with the sweet potatoes. Drizzle with olive oil and sprinkle with salt and pepper.
Remove the baking sheet from the oven and sprinkle the cheddar cheese over the broccoli and sweet potatoes.
Return the baking sheet to the oven and bake for an additional 5-10 minutes, or until the cheese is melted and bubbly.
Serve the baked sweet potatoes and broccoli hot.
Benefits: Sweet potatoes are high in vitamin A, vitamin C, and fibre, while broccoli is a good source of vitamin C, folate, and fibre. Cheddar cheese provides protein and calcium.

Nutrition Profile (per serving):
Calories: 296
Protein: 10g
Fat: 13g
Carbohydrates: 37g
Fibre: 7g

Salmon and Asparagus Foil Packets:

Ingredients:

2 salmon fillets
1 lb asparagus, trimmed
2 cloves garlic, minced
2 tablespoons olive oil
Salt and pepper to taste
Lemon slices for serving

Instructions:

Preheat the oven to 375°F (190°C).
Cut two large pieces of aluminium foil. Place half of the asparagus in the centre of each foil sheet.
Place a salmon fillet on top of each bed of asparagus. Sprinkle the garlic over the salmon and drizzle with olive oil. Season with salt and pepper.
Fold the edges of the foil up around the salmon and asparagus to form a packet. Make sure the packet is sealed tightly.
Place the packets on a baking sheet and bake for 15-20 minutes, or until the salmon is cooked through.
Carefully open the packets and serve hot, with lemon slices for squeezing over the salmon and asparagus.

Benefits: Salmon is a good source of protein and omega-3 fatty acids, while asparagus is a low-calorie vegetable that is high in folate, fiber, and vitamins A and C.

Nutrition Profile (per serving):
Calories: 375
Protein: 36g
Fat: 23g
Carbohydrates: 8g
Fiber: 4g

Lentil and Vegetable Stew:

Ingredients:

1 cup dry green lentils, rinsed and drained
1 can diced tomatoes, undrained
4 cups vegetable broth
2 large carrots, chopped
2 stalks celery, chopped
1 small onion, chopped
2 cloves garlic, minced
1 teaspoon dried thyme
Salt and pepper to taste

Instructions:

In a large pot, combine the lentils, diced tomatoes, vegetable broth, carrots, celery, onion, garlic, thyme, salt, and pepper.
Bring the mixture to a boil, then reduce heat to low and simmer for 30-40 minutes, or until the lentils are tender and the vegetables are cooked through.
Serve the lentil stew hot, with crusty bread or crackers.

Benefits: Lentils are a good source of protein and fibre, while vegetables provide important vitamins and minerals.

Nutrition Profile (per serving):
Calories: 251
Protein: 16g
Fat: 1g
Carbohydrates: 46g
Fibre: 17g

Chicken and Vegetable Stir Fry:

Ingredients:

1 lb boneless, skinless chicken breasts, sliced
2 cups broccoli florets
1 cup sliced bell peppers

1 small onion, sliced
2 cloves garlic, minced
2 tablespoons soy sauce
1 tablespoon cornstarch
2 tablespoons olive oil
Salt and pepper to taste
2 cups cooked brown rice

Instructions:

In a small bowl, whisk together the soy sauce and cornstarch until smooth.
In a large skillet or wok, heat the olive oil over high heat. Add the chicken and cook for 5-7 minutes, or until browned.
Add the broccoli, bell peppers, onion, and garlic to the skillet. Stir fry for 5-7 minutes, or until the vegetables are tender.
Pour the soy sauce mixture over the chicken and vegetables. Stir to combine and cook for 1-2 minutes, or until the sauce has thickened.
Serve the stir fry hot

Benefits: Chicken is a good source of protein, while vegetables provide important vitamins and minerals. Bell peppers are high in vitamin C, broccoli is a good source of fibre and vitamins A and C, and onions and garlic contain antioxidants.

Nutrition Profile (per serving, not including rice):
Calories: 313
Protein: 30g
Fat: 14g
Carbohydrates: 15g
Fibre: 4g

Note: The nutrition profile does not include the rice, which will add additional calories and carbohydrates to the dish.

Snacks and Desserts

As a pregnant woman, it is important to maintain a healthy and balanced diet for both you and your growing baby. This means including a variety of nutrient-rich foods, such as fruits, vegetables, whole grains, lean proteins, and healthy fats.

However, it is also okay to indulge in snacks and desserts in moderation. Eating a small portion of your favourite treat occasionally is unlikely to have a negative impact on your pregnancy, as long as it is part of an overall healthy diet.

It is important to note that excessive consumption of high-calorie, low-nutrient foods can contribute to excessive weight gain during pregnancy, which can increase the risk of complications such as gestational diabetes and high blood pressure. Therefore, it is important to maintain balance and moderation in your food choices.

As a pregnant woman, it's important to choose snacks and desserts that are nutritious and provide you and your baby with the essential nutrients you need. Here are some ideas:

Fresh fruits - Fruits are a great source of vitamins, fibre, and antioxidants. Try to incorporate a variety of fruits in your diet, such as berries, melons, apples, oranges, and bananas.

Nuts and seeds - Nuts and seeds are a good source of protein, healthy fats, and fibre. You can try almonds, walnuts, cashews, pumpkin seeds, or sunflower seeds.

Yogurt - Yogurt is a good source of calcium and probiotics, which are important for healthy digestion. You can choose low-fat or fat-free yoghourt and add fresh fruit or granola for extra flavour and texture.

Whole grain crackers - Whole grain crackers provide fibre and complex carbohydrates. You can pair them with hummus, cheese, or nut butter for added protein.

Dark chocolate - Dark chocolate is a good source of antioxidants and can be a satisfying dessert option in moderation. Aim for at least 70% cacao and limit your portion sizes.

Remember to choose snacks and desserts that are low in added sugars and avoid raw or undercooked animal products, like meat or eggs, to reduce the risk of foodborne illness.

Here are some snack and dessert recipes with instructions, benefits, and nutrition profile for you:

Greek Yoghourt with Berries and Granola

Ingredients:

1 cup Greek yoghourt
1/2 cup mixed berries (such as blueberries, raspberries, and strawberries)
1/4 cup granola

Instructions:

In a bowl, spoon the Greek yoghourt.
Add the mixed berries on top of the yoghourt.
Sprinkle the granola over the berries.
Enjoy!

Benefits: Greek yoghourt is a great source of calcium and protein, which are important for a growing baby's bones and muscles. Berries are high in antioxidants, fibre, and vitamin C, which can help support a healthy immune system. Granola provides healthy fats and fibre, which can help keep you full and satisfied.

Nutrition profile: 1 serving of this recipe provides approximately 237 calories, 16g protein, 27g carbohydrates, 7g fat, and 4g fibre.

Apple and Peanut Butter

Ingredients:

1 apple, sliced
2 tbsp peanut butter

Instructions:

Slice the apple into wedges.
Spread the peanut butter on top of the apple slices.
Enjoy!

Benefits: Apples are high in fibre, which can help prevent constipation during pregnancy. Peanut butter is a good source of protein and healthy fats, which can help support a healthy pregnancy.

Nutrition profile: 1 serving of this recipe provides approximately 210 calories, 5g protein, 26g carbohydrates, 11g fat, and 5g fiber.

Chocolate Avocado Pudding

Ingredients:

2 ripe avocados
1/2 cup unsweetened cocoa powder
1/2 cup maple syrup
1 tsp vanilla extract
1/4 cup almond milk

Instructions:

Cut the avocados in half and remove the pit.
Scoop out the flesh and place it in a food processor.
Add the cocoa powder, maple syrup, vanilla extract, and almond milk to the food processor.
Blend until smooth and creamy.
Serve immediately or chill in the refrigerator for later.

Benefits: Avocados are high in healthy fats, which can help support a healthy pregnancy. Cocoa powder is high in antioxidants, which can help protect against cell damage. Maple syrup is a natural sweetener that contains vitamins and minerals, such as zinc and manganese.

Nutrition profile: 1 serving of this recipe provides approximately 250 calories, 4g protein, 36g carbohydrates, 14g fat, and 9g fiber.

Hummus and Vegetables

Ingredients:

1/2 cup hummus
Assorted vegetables for dipping (such as carrots, celery, bell peppers, and cucumbers)

Instructions:

Place the hummus in a bowl.
Wash and chop the vegetables.
Serve the vegetables alongside the hummus for dipping.
Enjoy!

Benefits: Hummus is a good source of protein, fiber, and healthy fats, which can help support a healthy pregnancy. Vegetables are packed with vitamins, minerals, and antioxidants, which can help support a healthy immune system and prevent chronic diseases.

Nutrition profile: 1 serving of this recipe provides approximately 200 calories, 8g protein, 20g carbohydrates, 10g fat, and 8g fiber.

Banana and Almond Butter Toast

Ingredients:

1 slice of whole-grain bread
1 banana, sliced

1 tbsp almond butter

Instructions:

Toast the slice of bread.
Spread the almond butter on the toast.
Top with the sliced banana.
Enjoy!

Benefits: Whole-grain bread is high in fibre, which can help prevent constipation during pregnancy. Bananas are a good source of potassium and vitamin C, which can help support a healthy pregnancy. Almond butter is a good source of protein and healthy fats, which can help support a healthy pregnancy.

Nutrition profile: 1 serving of this recipe provides approximately 280 calories, 9g protein, 39g carbohydrates, 12g fat, and 7g fibre.

Berry Smoothie

Ingredients:

1 cup frozen mixed berries
1/2 cup plain Greek yoghourt
1/2 cup unsweetened almond milk
1 tbsp honey

Instructions:

Combine the frozen mixed berries, Greek yoghourt, almond milk, and honey in a blender.
Blend until smooth and creamy.
Pour into a glass and enjoy!

Benefits: Mixed berries are high in antioxidants, fibre, and vitamin C, which can help support a healthy immune system. Greek yoghourt is a good source of calcium and protein, which can help support a healthy pregnancy. Almond milk is a good source of calcium and vitamin D, which are important for bone health.

Nutrition profile: 1 serving of this recipe provides approximately 200 calories, 12g protein, 32g carbohydrates, 3g fat, and 6g fibre.

Roasted Chickpeas

Ingredients:

1 can of chickpeas, drained and rinsed
1 tbsp olive oil
1 tsp paprika
1 tsp garlic powder
Salt to taste

Instructions:

Preheat the oven to 400°F (200°C).
Rinse and drain the chickpeas.
Spread the chickpeas on a baking sheet.
Drizzle with olive oil and sprinkle with paprika, garlic powder, and salt.
Toss to coat evenly.
Bake for 20-30 minutes, or until crispy.
Enjoy!

Benefits: Chickpeas are a good source of protein, fibre, and folate, which can help support a healthy pregnancy. Olive oil is a good source of healthy fats, which can help support a healthy pregnancy. Paprika and garlic powder are flavorful spices that can add variety to your diet.

Nutrition profile: 1 serving of this recipe provides approximately 165 calories, 6g protein, 20g carbohydrates, 7g fat, and 6g fibre.

Apple Oatmeal Cookies

Ingredients:

2 cups old-fashioned oats
1 cup whole-wheat flour
1/2 cup unsweetened applesauce
1/4 cup honey
1/4 cup coconut oil
1 egg
1 tsp baking powder
1 tsp cinnamon
1/2 tsp salt
1 apple, grated

Instructions:

Preheat the oven to 350°F (180°C).
In a bowl, combine the oats, flour, baking powder, cinnamon, and salt.
In a separate bowl, whisk together the applesauce, honey, coconut oil, and egg.
Add the wet ingredients to the dry ingredients and mix well.
Fold in the grated apple.
Drop spoonfuls of the mixture onto a baking sheet.
Bake for 12-15 minutes, or until lightly golden.
Enjoy!

Benefits: Oats are a good source of fiber, which can help prevent constipation during pregnancy. Whole-wheat flour is a good source of fiber and B vitamins, which can help support a healthy pregnancy. Applesauce and honey provide natural sweetness without added sugar, which can help reduce the risk of gestational diabetes.

Nutrition profile: 1 serving of this recipe (2 cookies) provides approximately 170 calories, 4g protein, 26g carbohydrates, 6g fat, and 3g fiber.

Chocolate Chia Pudding

Ingredients:

1/4 cup chia seeds
1 cup unsweetened almond milk
1 tbsp honey
1 tbsp unsweetened cocoa powder
1/2 tsp vanilla extract

Instructions:

In a bowl, whisk together the chia seeds, almond milk, honey, cocoa powder, and vanilla extract.
Let the mixture sit for 10-15 minutes, or until thickened.
Serve immediately or chill in the refrigerator for later.
Enjoy!

Benefits: Chia seeds are a good source of fiber, protein, and omega-3 fatty acids, which can help support a healthy pregnancy. Almond milk is a good source of calcium and vitamin D, which are important for bone health. Cocoa powder is high in antioxidants, which can help protect against cell damage.

Nutrition profile: 1 serving of this recipe provides approximately 180 calories, 6g protein, 22g carbohydrates,

Greek Yoghourt Parfait

Ingredients:

1 cup plain Greek yoghourt
1/2 cup fresh berries (such as strawberries, blueberries, or raspberries)
1/4 cup granola
1 tbsp honey

Instructions:

In a bowl, layer the Greek yoghourt, fresh berries, and granola.
Drizzle with honey.
Enjoy!

Benefits: Greek yoghourt is a good source of protein and calcium, which are important for foetal development. Berries are high in antioxidants and vitamin C, which can help support a healthy pregnancy. Granola provides fibre and healthy fats, which can help prevent constipation and support a healthy pregnancy.

Nutrition profile: 1 serving of this recipe provides approximately 280 calories, 19g protein, 39g carbohydrates, 6g fat, and 5g fibre.

Sweet Potato Fries

Ingredients:

2 sweet potatoes, peeled and sliced into thin wedges
1 tbsp olive oil
1 tsp paprika
1 tsp garlic powder
Salt to taste

Instructions:

Preheat the oven to 400°F (200°C).
In a bowl, toss the sweet potato wedges with olive oil, paprika, garlic powder, and salt.
Spread the sweet potato wedges on a baking sheet.
Bake for 20-30 minutes, or until crispy.
Enjoy!

Benefits: Sweet potatoes are high in fibre, vitamin A, and potassium, which can help support a healthy pregnancy. Olive oil is a good source of healthy fats, which can help support a healthy pregnancy. Paprika and garlic powder are flavorful spices that can add variety to your diet.

Nutrition profile: 1 serving of this recipe provides approximately 200 calories, 2g protein, 32g carbohydrates, 7g fat, and 5g fibre.

Banana Bread Muffins

Ingredients:

2 ripe bananas, mashed
1/3 cup coconut oil
1/4 cup honey
1 egg
1 tsp vanilla extract
1 1/2 cups whole-wheat flour
1 tsp baking powder
1/2 tsp baking soda
1/2 tsp cinnamon
1/4 tsp salt

Instructions:

Preheat the oven to 350°F (180°C).
In a bowl, mix together the mashed bananas, coconut oil, honey, egg, and vanilla extract.
In a separate bowl, mix together the whole-wheat flour, baking powder, baking soda, cinnamon, and salt.
Add the wet ingredients to the dry ingredients and mix well.
Divide the mixture evenly into a muffin tin.
Bake for 15-20 minutes, or until lightly golden.
Enjoy!

Benefits: Bananas are high in potassium, which can help regulate blood pressure during pregnancy. Coconut oil provides healthy fats, which can help support a healthy pregnancy. Whole-wheat flour is a good source of fibre and B vitamins, which can help support a healthy pregnancy.

Nutrition profile: 1 serving of this recipe (1 muffin) provides approximately 180 calories, 3g protein, 27g carbohydrates, 7g fat, and 3g fibre.

I hope these recipes and their nutritional benefits help you make healthy choices during your pregnancy!

Smoothies and Juices

Smoothies and juices can be a healthy addition to a pregnant woman's diet, providing essential nutrients and hydration. Here are some ideas for smoothies and juices that are safe and nutritious for pregnant women:

Green smoothie: Blend together spinach, kale, banana, pineapple, and coconut water for a nutrient-packed drink.

Carrot and ginger juice: Juice fresh carrots and ginger for a refreshing and immune-boosting drink.

Mango lassi: Blend mango, yogurt, and honey for a creamy and delicious drink that's rich in calcium and vitamin C.

Berry smoothie: Blend mixed berries, Greek yogurt, and honey for a sweet and tangy drink that's high in antioxidants and protein.

Watermelon juice: Juice fresh watermelon for a hydrating and refreshing drink that's packed with vitamin C.

Banana and almond butter smoothie: Blend banana, almond butter, almond milk, and honey for a protein-packed drink that's perfect for a quick breakfast.

Pineapple and coconut smoothie: Blend pineapple, coconut milk, and vanilla for a tropical drink that's high in potassium and fibre.

Beet and apple juice: Juice fresh beets, apples, and carrots for a nutrient-packed drink that's high in iron and vitamin C.

Avocado smoothie: Blend avocado, Greek yoghourt, spinach, and honey for a creamy and filling drink that's rich in healthy fats and protein.

Orange and carrot smoothie: Blend fresh orange juice, carrots, and ginger for a refreshing drink that's high in vitamin A and antioxidants.

Blueberry and banana smoothie: Blend frozen blueberries, banana, almond milk, and honey for a sweet and satisfying drink that's packed with fibre and vitamin C.

Cucumber and mint juice: Juice fresh cucumbers and mint for a hydrating and refreshing drink that's perfect for a hot day.

Chocolate and banana smoothie: Blend banana, almond milk, cocoa powder, and honey for a decadent and satisfying drink that's high in potassium and antioxidants.

Strawberry and kiwi smoothie: Blend fresh strawberries, kiwi, Greek yoghourt, and honey for a sweet and tangy drink that's packed with vitamin C and protein.

Remember to always wash fruits and vegetables thoroughly before using them in smoothies and juices.

It's important to remember that pregnant women should avoid unpasteurized juices, which can contain harmful bacteria. It's also important to consult with a healthcare provider about any dietary concerns or restrictions during pregnancy.

It's also important to consult with a healthcare provider about any dietary concerns or restrictions during pregnancy.

Chapter 4: Addressing Specific Pregnancy-Related Concerns with Real Food

Pregnancy is a time of great excitement and anticipation for most women, but it can also be a time of concern and worry. There are many factors to consider during pregnancy, including proper nutrition and diet. Eating a healthy diet during pregnancy is essential for both the mother and the developing baby. Real food can play a significant role in addressing specific pregnancy-related concerns.

One of the main concerns during pregnancy is gestational diabetes. This type of diabetes occurs during pregnancy and can cause complications for both the mother and the baby. A diet high in real, whole foods can help manage blood sugar levels and prevent gestational diabetes. Whole foods, such as fruits, vegetables, and whole grains, contain complex carbohydrates that are slowly digested, keeping blood sugar levels stable. Additionally, real food sources of protein, such as beans, lentils, and lean meats, can also help stabilise blood sugar levels.

Another concern during pregnancy is pre-eclampsia, a condition characterised by high blood pressure and protein in the urine. Pre-eclampsia can be dangerous for both the mother and the baby, and real food can help manage this condition. Eating a diet rich in potassium, magnesium, and calcium can help lower blood pressure and reduce the risk of pre-eclampsia. Real food sources of these nutrients include leafy greens, nuts and seeds, dairy products, and whole grains.

Iron-deficiency anaemia is also a concern during pregnancy, as the developing baby requires iron for proper growth and development. Real food sources of iron, such as lean meats, beans, lentils, and leafy greens, can help prevent anaemia. Eating foods rich in vitamin C, such as citrus fruits, bell peppers, and broccoli, can also help the body absorb iron more efficiently.

Finally, many women experience morning sickness during pregnancy, which can make it challenging to eat a healthy diet. Real food sources of ginger, such as ginger tea or ginger chews, can help alleviate nausea and improve digestion. Additionally, eating small, frequent meals throughout the day can help manage morning sickness and ensure proper nutrition.

Let's dive in more for a more broad knowledge

Gestational Diabetes

Gestational diabetes mellitus (GDM) is a condition characterised by high blood sugar levels during pregnancy. It usually develops around the 24th to 28th week of pregnancy, and it affects approximately 10% of pregnant women. GDM can have serious consequences for both the mother and the baby if left untreated.

Causes of Gestational Diabetes:

GDM is caused by the hormonal changes that occur during pregnancy. As the pregnancy progresses, the placenta produces more hormones that can interfere with the action of insulin, a hormone that regulates blood sugar levels. Insulin helps glucose (a type of sugar) move from the bloodstream into the body's cells, where it is used as energy. However, when insulin is not working properly, glucose levels in the bloodstream remain high, leading to GDM.

Risk factors for developing GDM include being overweight or obese before pregnancy, having a family history of diabetes, being older than 25 years, having previously given birth to a baby weighing over 4 kilograms (8 pounds 13 ounces), and having polycystic ovary syndrome (PCOS).

Effects of Gestational Diabetes on the Mother:

Women with GDM are at increased risk of developing preeclampsia (a potentially life-threatening condition that causes high blood pressure and damage to organs), having a caesarean delivery, and developing type 2 diabetes later in life.

Effects of Gestational Diabetes on the Baby:

Babies born to mothers with GDM are at risk of being large for their gestational age, having a low blood sugar level at birth, and being born prematurely. These babies are also at increased risk of developing type 2 diabetes and obesity later in life.

Prevention and Treatment of Gestational Diabetes:

While GDM cannot be completely prevented, there are ways to reduce the risk of developing it. Maintaining a healthy weight before and during pregnancy, eating a healthy diet that is low in sugar and refined carbohydrates, and staying physically active can all help to reduce the risk of GDM.

If GDM is diagnosed, it is important to manage it carefully to prevent complications. This may involve making dietary changes, such as eating smaller, more frequent meals that are low in sugar and high in fibre, and getting regular exercise. In some cases, medication, such as insulin injections, may be necessary to control blood sugar levels.

Regular prenatal care is essential for the early detection and management of GDM. Pregnant women should be screened for GDM between 24 and 28 weeks of pregnancy, and earlier if they have risk factors for GDM. After delivery, women with GDM should continue to have their blood sugar levels monitored to ensure that they do not develop type 2 diabetes.

In conclusion, Gestational diabetes is a serious condition that can have significant consequences for both the mother and the baby if left untreated. While it cannot be completely prevented, maintaining a healthy lifestyle before and during pregnancy and receiving regular prenatal care can help to reduce the risk of developing GDM and ensure that it is managed effectively.

Morning Sickness

Morning sickness is a common condition that affects many pregnant women, usually during the first trimester of pregnancy. It is characterised by feelings of nausea, vomiting, and sometimes dizziness or fatigue. The exact causes of morning sickness are not well understood, but it is believed to be related to hormonal changes in the body, particularly the increase in levels of human chorionic gonadotropin (hCG) and oestrogen.

While morning sickness is a normal part of pregnancy, severe or prolonged cases can have negative effects on both the mother and the developing foetus. For the mother, severe vomiting and dehydration can lead to weight loss, nutritional deficiencies, and electrolyte imbalances. For the foetus, maternal dehydration can result in decreased blood flow to the placenta, which can affect foetal growth and development.

There are several ways to manage and prevent morning sickness. Some tips include:

Eat small, frequent meals: Eating small, frequent meals throughout the day can help keep your blood sugar levels stable and prevent nausea.

Avoid trigger foods: Certain foods, such as spicy or greasy foods, can trigger nausea and vomiting. Avoid these foods and stick to bland, easy-to-digest foods like crackers, rice, and chicken broth.

Stay hydrated: Dehydration can make morning sickness worse, so it's important to stay hydrated. Sip on water, ginger tea, or other clear fluids throughout the day.

Get plenty of rest: Fatigue can exacerbate morning sickness, so make sure you're getting plenty of rest and sleep.

Consider medication: If your morning sickness is severe, your doctor may prescribe medication to help manage your symptoms.

Try alternative therapies: Some women find relief from morning sickness through alternative therapies such as acupuncture, acupressure, or aromatherapy.

It's important to remember that every woman's experience with morning sickness is different, and what works for one woman may not work for another. If you're struggling with morning sickness, talk to your healthcare provider to find the best approach for managing your symptoms.

Anaemia

Anaemia is a common condition among pregnant women, and it occurs when the body does not have enough healthy red blood cells to carry oxygen to the tissues and organs. Anaemia can have serious effects on both the mother and the developing foetus.

Causes of Anaemia in Pregnant Women:

Iron deficiency: This is the most common cause of anaemia in pregnant women, and it occurs when the body doesn't have enough iron to produce haemoglobin.
Folate deficiency: Folate is a B vitamin that is important for the production of new cells. A deficiency in folate can lead to anaemia.
Vitamin B12 deficiency: This vitamin is necessary for the production of red blood cells, and a deficiency can lead to anaemia.
Blood loss: Heavy menstrual bleeding or bleeding during pregnancy or childbirth can lead to anaemia.
Other medical conditions: Certain medical conditions like sickle cell anaemia and thalassemia can cause anaemia.
Effects of Anaemia on Pregnant Women:

Fatigue and weakness
Shortness of breath
Dizziness or fainting
Increased risk of infections
Preterm birth
Low birth weight
Maternal mortality
Effects of Anaemia on the Developing Foetus:

Low birth weight
Premature birth
Developmental delays
Increased risk of infections
How to Avoid Anaemia During Pregnancy:

Eat a healthy and balanced diet rich in iron, folate, and vitamin B12.
Good sources of iron include red meat, poultry, fish, beans, lentils,
spinach, and fortified cereals. Good sources of folate include leafy green
vegetables, citrus fruits, beans, and fortified cereals. Good sources of
vitamin B12 include meat, poultry, fish, and dairy products.
Take prenatal vitamins as prescribed by your healthcare provider.
Avoid drinking tea or coffee with meals, as these can inhibit the
absorption of iron from food.
Avoid consuming calcium-rich foods like dairy products and
supplements at the same time as iron-rich foods or supplements, as
calcium can also inhibit the absorption of iron.
Treat any medical conditions that can cause anaemia.
Manage heavy menstrual bleeding or bleeding during pregnancy or
childbirth.
Discuss the possibility of iron supplements with your healthcare provider
if you are at risk of developing anaemia or if you are already anemic.
It is important to diagnose and treat anaemia during pregnancy to
prevent any adverse effects on both the mother and the developing
foetus. If you are experiencing symptoms of anaemia or are at risk of
developing anaemia during pregnancy, please consult your healthcare
provider.

Constipation

Constipation is a common problem among pregnant women due to
hormonal changes and physical pressure on the digestive tract. Here are
some causes and effects of constipation in pregnant women, as well as
tips on how to avoid it:

Causes of constipation in pregnant women:

Hormonal changes: During pregnancy, there is an increase in the hormone progesterone, which can relax the muscles in the intestines and slow down digestion.

Pressure on the digestive tract: As the uterus grows, it can put pressure on the digestive tract, making it harder for food to move through the intestines.

Iron supplements: Pregnant women may be advised to take iron supplements, which can cause constipation.

Effects of constipation in pregnant women:

Discomfort and pain: Constipation can cause discomfort and pain in the lower abdomen.

Haemorrhoids: Straining during bowel movements can increase the risk of developing haemorrhoids, which are swollen veins in the rectum or anus.

Anal fissures: Constipation can also cause small tears in the lining of the anus, which can be painful.

Tips to avoid constipation in pregnant women:

Drink plenty of water: Staying hydrated can help soften stools and make them easier to pass.

Eat a high-fibre diet: Eating foods high in fibre, such as fruits, vegetables, and whole grains, can help keep the digestive system regular.

Exercise regularly: Regular exercise can help keep the digestive system moving and prevent constipation.

Take stool softeners: If constipation persists, your doctor may recommend a stool softener or laxative that is safe for pregnant women.

Talk to your doctor: If you are experiencing constipation, talk to your doctor about possible treatment options and ways to manage the condition during pregnancy.

Heartburn

Heartburn is a common condition experienced by many pregnant women, especially during the second and third trimesters. It is caused by the stomach acid that flows back up into the oesophagus, causing a burning sensation in the chest and throat. The following are some of the causes and effects of heartburn during pregnancy:

Causes:

Hormonal changes: During pregnancy, the hormone progesterone relaxes the muscles of the digestive system, which can cause the stomach acid to flow back up into the oesophagus.
Pressure on the stomach: As the baby grows, it can put pressure on the stomach, causing the stomach acid to move up into the oesophagus.
Eating large meals: Consuming large meals can increase the risk of heartburn during pregnancy.
Effects:

Discomfort and pain: Heartburn during pregnancy can cause discomfort and pain in the chest and throat.
Difficulty sleeping: Pregnant women who experience heartburn may have difficulty sleeping, which can lead to fatigue and other pregnancy-related issues.
Dental problems: Stomach acid that flows into the mouth can cause dental problems such as erosion of the enamel and tooth decay.
How to avoid heartburn during pregnancy:

Eat smaller meals throughout the day instead of three large meals.
Avoid eating spicy or acidic foods that can trigger heartburn.
Wait at least two hours after eating before lying down or going to bed.
Avoid drinking large amounts of fluids with meals.

Wear loose-fitting clothing that doesn't put pressure on the stomach.
Elevate the head of the bed by 6-8 inches to prevent stomach acid from
flowing back up into the oesophagus while sleeping.
If heartburn persists despite these measures, pregnant women should
speak with their healthcare provider for additional advice and treatment
options.

In conclusion, addressing specific pregnancy-related concerns with real
food is crucial for the health of both the mother and the baby. Eating a
nutritious diet during pregnancy can help to prevent complications such
as gestational diabetes, pre-eclampsia, and low birth weight.

By focusing on real, whole foods, pregnant women can ensure that they
are getting the necessary nutrients and avoiding potentially harmful
substances such as artificial sweeteners, preservatives, and pesticides.
Additionally, choosing foods that are high in fibre and low in added
sugars can help to regulate blood sugar levels and prevent excessive
weight gain.

For those dealing with pregnancy-related concerns at the moment, it is
important to consult with a healthcare professional to determine the best
course of action. A registered dietitian can provide personalised nutrition
advice and help to create a meal plan that meets individual needs and
preferences.

Ultimately, by making smart food choices and incorporating a variety of
nutrient-dense foods into their diets, pregnant women can support a
healthy pregnancy and give their babies the best possible start in life.

Chapter 5: Beyond Pregnancy: Real Food Nutrition for Postpartum Recovery

Postpartum refers to the period of time following childbirth, typically the first six weeks after delivery. This period is often referred to as the "fourth trimester" because it is a time of significant physical and emotional changes for both the mother and the baby.

In this chapter, we will be discussing the importance of real food nutrition for postpartum recovery. Many new mothers focus solely on the health of their baby and may neglect their own nutritional needs, but proper nutrition is critical for the healing and recovery process after childbirth. We will explore the specific nutrient needs of postpartum women and provide practical tips for incorporating real, whole foods into the diet to support optimal recovery and long-term health.

Nourishing Foods for Postpartum Healing

The postpartum period is a time of physical and emotional healing for new mothers. It is important for women to consume nourishing foods during this time to support their recovery and provide essential nutrients for breastfeeding.

Here are some nourishing foods that can help with postpartum healing:

Protein-rich foods: Protein is essential for tissue repair and growth. Good sources of protein include eggs, lean meats, poultry, fish, beans, lentils, and tofu.

Leafy greens: Leafy greens are packed with vitamins and minerals, including iron, calcium, and vitamin K. These nutrients can help with healing and support bone health. Examples of leafy greens include spinach, kale, collard greens, and Swiss chard.

Whole grains: Whole grains are rich in fiber, B vitamins, and minerals such as iron and zinc. Good sources of whole grains include brown rice, quinoa, whole wheat bread, and oatmeal.

Fatty fish: Fatty fish such as salmon, sardines, and mackerel are rich in omega-3 fatty acids, which can help with inflammation and support brain health.

Nuts and seeds: Nuts and seeds are a good source of healthy fats, protein, and minerals such as magnesium and zinc. Examples include almonds, walnuts, chia seeds, and flaxseeds.

Fruits and vegetables: Fruits and vegetables are packed with vitamins, minerals, and fibre. Eating a variety of colourful fruits and vegetables can provide a range of nutrients to support healing and overall health.

Bone broth: Bone broth is made by simmering animal bones and connective tissue in water. It is rich in minerals such as calcium, magnesium, and phosphorus, as well as collagen, which can support gut health and joint health.

Herbal teas: Herbal teas such as chamomile, ginger, and peppermint can be soothing and help with digestion.

Adequate hydration: It is important for new mothers to stay hydrated during the postpartum period, especially if they are breastfeeding. Drinking enough water and other fluids can help with milk production, prevent constipation, and support overall health.

Iron-rich foods: Many women experience iron deficiency anaemia after giving birth, so it is important to consume iron-rich foods such as red meat, poultry, beans, lentils, leafy greens, and fortified cereals.

Healthy fats: Consuming healthy fats such as those found in nuts, seeds, fatty fish, and avocado can provide essential fatty acids for brain development in the baby and support hormone balance in the mother.

Avoidance of highly processed foods: Highly processed foods such as sugary snacks, fast food, and refined grains can be low in nutrients and contribute to inflammation in the body. It is best to avoid these types of foods and instead focus on whole, nutrient-dense foods.

Slow and steady weight loss: While it is common for new mothers to want to lose their pregnancy weight quickly, it is important to approach weight loss slowly and gradually to avoid negatively impacting milk supply and overall health. A registered dietitian can help new mothers develop a healthy and sustainable meal plan to support weight loss goals while still meeting nutrient needs.

Mindful eating: The postpartum period can be a stressful and busy time, but it is important to prioritise self-care and mindful eating. Taking the time to sit down and enjoy meals, listening to hunger and fullness cues, and avoiding distractions such as screens can help with digestion and overall well-being.

Supplements: Some women may require supplements such as iron, vitamin D, or omega-3 fatty acids to meet their nutrient needs during the postpartum period. Consulting with a healthcare professional or registered dietitian can help determine if supplements are necessary and what types and dosages are appropriate.

It is important for new mothers to prioritise self-care during the postpartum period, including nourishing foods and adequate rest. Consultation with a healthcare professional or a registered dietitian can provide personalised recommendations for optimal postpartum nutrition.

Meal Planning for Postpartum

Postpartum meal planning is an essential aspect of postpartum care that focuses on providing the necessary nutrients and support for new mothers during the first few weeks after giving birth. This period is often referred to as the "fourth trimester" and is a critical time for recovery, physical healing, and adjusting to life with a new baby. Proper nutrition during this time can help support physical recovery, energy levels, and emotional well-being.

Postpartum meal planning typically involves preparing and planning meals and snacks that are nutrient-dense and easy to digest, as the body requires extra energy and nutrients to heal and produce breast milk. Some examples of nutrient-dense foods that are often included in postpartum meal planning include leafy greens, whole grains, lean proteins, healthy fats, and fruits and vegetables.

In addition to focusing on nutrient-dense foods, postpartum meal planning may also involve preparing meals and snacks in advance to make mealtime easier during the busy and often overwhelming postpartum period. Meal prepping and planning can help new mothers ensure they have healthy meals and snacks on hand, even when they are short on time or energy.

Overall, postpartum meal planning is an essential aspect of postpartum care that can help support physical and emotional recovery during the fourth trimester. By focusing on nutrient-dense foods and making mealtime easier and more manageable, new mothers can prioritise their health and well-being as they adjust to life with a new baby.

Recipes for Postpartum Recovery

Postpartum recovery is an essential part of a new mother's journey, as the body undergoes many changes during pregnancy and childbirth. Here are some nutritious and healing recipes that can aid in postpartum recovery:

Nourishing Bone Broth: Bone broth is a great source of essential nutrients that can help restore and repair the body after childbirth. To make bone broth, simmer chicken or beef bones for several hours with vegetables and herbs.

Quinoa Salad: Quinoa is a high-protein grain that is easy to digest and packed with nutrients. Combine cooked quinoa with chopped vegetables, herbs, and a simple dressing for a nourishing salad.

Salmon and Sweet Potato Hash: Salmon is a great source of omega-3 fatty acids, which are important for postpartum healing. Combine cooked salmon with roasted sweet potatoes, sautéed vegetables, and herbs for a hearty and nutritious meal.

Greek Yogurt and Fruit Parfait: Greek yoghourt is high in protein and calcium, which can help with postpartum recovery. Layer Greek yoghourt with fresh fruit and granola for a delicious and healthy breakfast or snack.

Oatmeal with Nuts and Berries: Oatmeal is a great source of fibre and can help regulate digestion after childbirth. Top cooked oatmeal with chopped nuts, fresh berries, and a drizzle of honey for a delicious and nutritious breakfast.

Turmeric Ginger Tea: Turmeric and ginger are anti-inflammatory and can help with postpartum healing. Boil water with turmeric and ginger, then strain and add honey and lemon for a soothing and healing tea.

Lentil Soup: Lentils are an excellent source of plant-based protein, fibre, and iron, which can help with postpartum recovery. Make a hearty lentil soup with vegetables and herbs for a comforting and nutritious meal.

Green Smoothie: A green smoothie is a great way to pack in nutrients and support postpartum healing. Blend together spinach, kale, banana, almond milk, and a scoop of protein powder for a delicious and nutrient-dense smoothie.

Chicken and Vegetable Stir-Fry: Stir-fries are quick and easy to make and can be packed with nutritious ingredients. Sauté chicken with colourful vegetables like bell peppers, carrots, and broccoli, then season with ginger, garlic, and soy sauce for a tasty and healthy meal.

Baked Sweet Potato with Black Beans and Avocado: Sweet potatoes are a great source of fibre and antioxidants, which can help with postpartum healing. Bake a sweet potato, then top it with black beans, avocado, and a squeeze of lime for a delicious and nourishing meal.

Chia Seed Pudding: Chia seeds are high in omega-3 fatty acids and fibre, which can help with postpartum healing. Mix chia seeds with almond milk, honey, and vanilla extract, then refrigerate overnight for a delicious and nutritious pudding.

Spinach and Feta Stuffed Chicken Breasts: Chicken is a great source of protein, and adding spinach and feta cheese makes it even more nutritious. Stuff chicken breasts with the spinach and feta mixture, then bake for a delicious and healthy meal.

Berry Smoothie Bowl: Smoothie bowls are a great way to pack in nutrients and can be customised to your liking. Blend together frozen berries, banana, almond milk, and a scoop of protein powder, then top with granola and fresh berries for a satisfying breakfast or snack.

Roasted Vegetable Quiche: Quiche is a versatile dish that can be packed with vegetables and protein. Roast vegetables like bell peppers, zucchini, and mushrooms, then add them to an egg and milk mixture with cheese and herbs. Bake for a nutritious and delicious meal.

Coconut Curry with Shrimp and Vegetables: Coconut curry is a flavorful and nourishing dish that can be customised with your favourite protein and vegetables. Sauté shrimp and vegetables like bell peppers and broccoli, then add coconut milk and curry paste for a delicious and healthy meal.

Overnight Oats with Nut Butter and Banana: Overnight oats are a convenient and nutritious breakfast option. Mix oats with almond milk, nut butter, honey, and banana, then refrigerate overnight for a delicious and satisfying breakfast.

Baked Salmon with Asparagus: Salmon is a great source of omega-3 fatty acids, which can help with postpartum healing. Roast salmon and asparagus with herbs and lemon for a healthy and delicious meal.

Quinoa and Veggie Stir-Fry: Quinoa is a nutritious grain that can be used in a variety of dishes. Sauté quinoa with mixed vegetables like carrots, peas, and bell peppers, then season with soy sauce and sesame oil for a flavorful and healthy stir-fry.

Sweet Potato and Black Bean Enchiladas: Sweet potatoes and black beans are both nutritious and delicious. Stuff tortillas with sweet potatoes, black beans, and cheese, then bake with enchilada sauce for a comforting and healthy meal.

Green Lentil Salad: Green lentils are a great source of protein, fibre, and iron, which can support postpartum recovery. Mix cooked lentils with chopped vegetables like bell peppers, cucumber, and cherry tomatoes, then dress with lemon and olive oil for a refreshing and nourishing salad.

Banana and Almond Butter Smoothie: Bananas are high in potassium, which can help regulate blood pressure and support postpartum healing. Blend banana with almond butter, almond milk, and a scoop of protein powder for a delicious and nutritious smoothie.
The postpartum recovery recipes mentioned earlier are beneficial in several ways:

They are nutrient-dense: The recipes are rich in nutrients like protein, fibre, healthy fats, vitamins, and minerals. These nutrients are essential for postpartum recovery, as they support healing, boost energy, and promote overall health.

They support lactation: Many of the recipes are also lactation-friendly, meaning they can help boost milk production and supply. For example, foods like oats, salmon, lentils, and leafy greens are known to be galactagogues, which can support milk production.

They are easy to digest: The recipes are made with whole, minimally processed ingredients that are easy to digest and gentle on the digestive system. This is important during the postpartum period, as the body is still recovering and adjusting to changes.

They promote overall health: The recipes are balanced and nourishing, which can promote overall health and wellbeing. Eating a variety of nutrient-dense foods can support the immune system, reduce inflammation, and promote mental health.

Overall, these postpartum recovery recipes can help support postpartum recovery, boost energy and milk production, and promote overall health and wellbeing. It's important to prioritise nourishing and healing foods during the postpartum period to support your recovery and overall health.

Conclusion: Embracing a Real Food Lifestyle for a Healthy Pregnancy and Beyond

Pregnancy is an exciting and transformative time in a woman's life, but it can also be overwhelming, confusing, and challenging. With so much conflicting information about what to eat and what to avoid, it's easy to feel lost in the sea of dietary advice. However, there is one fundamental principle that underpins all good nutrition: eat real food.

A real food lifestyle is centred on whole, unprocessed, nutrient-dense foods that nourish your body and support optimal health. This means choosing fresh fruits and vegetables, whole grains, grass-fed meats, wild-caught fish, pastured eggs, nuts and seeds, and healthy fats like avocado, coconut oil, and olive oil. It also means avoiding highly processed and refined foods, sugary drinks, artificial sweeteners, and other empty calories that provide little nutrition and can be harmful to both you and your baby.

Embracing a real food lifestyle during pregnancy has numerous benefits. First and foremost, it ensures that you are getting the essential nutrients your body needs to support a healthy pregnancy and foetal development. These nutrients include protein, healthy fats, folate, iron, calcium, vitamin D, and omega-3 fatty acids, among others. Eating real food also helps regulate your blood sugar, reduce inflammation, and support your immune system, which can help prevent complications like gestational diabetes, pre-eclampsia, and infections.

But the benefits of a real food lifestyle don't end with pregnancy. Eating a diet rich in whole foods can also help you recover more quickly after childbirth, support lactation and breastfeeding, and reduce your risk of chronic diseases like diabetes, heart disease, and cancer. Plus, it sets a positive example for your children and helps instil healthy habits that can last a lifetime.

Of course, transitioning to a real food lifestyle can be daunting, especially if you're used to relying on convenience foods and processed snacks.

However, making small changes over time can add up to big improvements in your health and well-being. Start by incorporating more whole foods into your diet, cooking at home more often, and reducing your intake of sugary drinks and snacks. Experiment with new recipes and flavours, and don't be afraid to ask for help or support from a registered dietitian or other healthcare provider.

In conclusion, a real food lifestyle is not just a fad or a trend; it's a sustainable, evidence-based approach to nourishing yourself and your family. By choosing whole, unprocessed foods and avoiding harmful additives and chemicals, you can support a healthy pregnancy, a vibrant postpartum period, and a lifetime of optimal health and well-being. So take the first step today and start nourishing your body with the real food it deserves.

"From morning sickness to motherhood, a real food lifestyle is the recipe for a healthy and happy pregnancy. So ditch the processed junk, embrace whole foods, and nourish yourself and your baby for a lifetime of wellness!"

www.ingramcontent.com/pod-product-compliance
Lightning Source LLC
Chambersburg PA
CBHW050831250726
48653CB00006B/2547